Effective Treatment for Stress and Anxiety

By
Lynne D M Noble

Copyright 2018 Lynne D M Noble

This book shall not, by way of trade or otherwise, be lent, re-sold, hired out, or otherwise circulated without the prior consent of the copyright holder or the publisher in any form of binding or cover than that in which it is published and without a similar condition including this condition being imposed on the subsequent purchaser.
The use of its contents in another media is also subject to the same conditions.

Independently published

Contents

Preface	Page V
The fight or flight response	Page 1
External cause of stress	Page 10
The naturally anxious person	Page 12
Treatment for Anxiety, stress and depression	Page 14
The importance of neurotransmitters in mental health	Page 42
Glycine; anti-anxiolytic	Page 56
Phenylalanine	Page 65
Low Potassium and Magnesium	Page 68
Altered pH; Altered mental state	Page 78
The B vitamins	Page 92
Vanadium toxicity, biotin and iron deficiency	Page 107

Dedication

This book is dedicated to all who suffer from anxiety and depression and especially to those many members of my family for whom it has been a life-long companion. And especially for my son

Dylan

1972-1997

Acknowledgement

Many thanks to all my friends who have supplied the inspiration to write this book. If nothing else, I have learned that depression and anxiety escape no one and manifests itself in many different ways. For some it is but a fleeting companion and for others it is lifelong.

For some, it inspires them to write music and poetry and to reach into the depths of their souls. For others, it is overwhelming and only the solitude of a dark and silent room offers them any comfort.

Some cry easily and others are given to anger or indifference. There are few that would wish this on their worst enemy.

So, I thank you all for sharing your stories with me.

About the Author

Lynne Noble was born in 1953 in Huddersfield, West Yorkshire. From a very early age, Lynne showed an interest in nutrition and genetics avidly reading any books that she could get her hands on at the time.

Initially, Lynne studied orthopaedics but events led her to work with the elderly mentally infirm. Here, her interest in neurodegenerative disorders and pain syndromes developed.

Lynne undertook rigorous programmes of study, completing her Cert Ed., (FE) BSc (Hons) and Adv. Dip Education simultaneously before moving onto her M.Ed.

From there she took further demanding programmes in Human Nutrition, Pharmacology, Neuroscience, Genetics and Immunology. During this time, she was given many prestigious awards for her academic work. It was noted then that Lynne was not afraid of tackling difficult subjects.

She began her law degree but ill health prevented her from pursuing this. However, in this time, she moved from being a foster parent to adoptive parent.

She has been instrumental in setting up projects in the community for disadvantaged groups.

She is a member of the Guild of Health Writers and the British Union of Journalists.

Now retired, she lives with her husband in a historic Georgian riverside town in the West Midlands. She enjoys gardening, watching her husband bowling and researching.

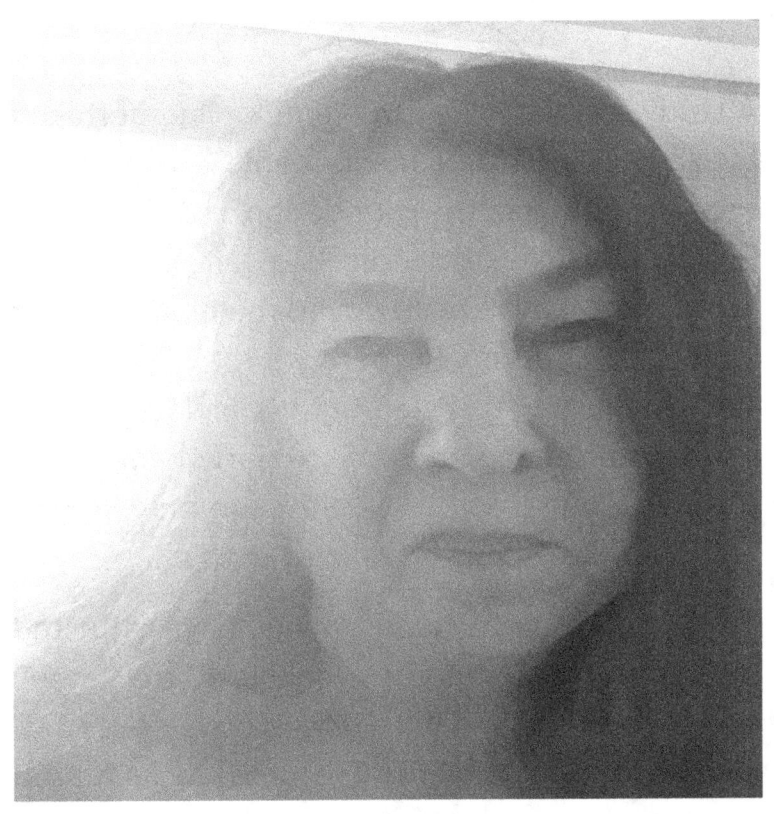

Author Lynne Noble at home aged 67 yrs.

Preface

A study conducted by an online poll undertaken by YouGov of 4,169 respondents on behalf of the Mental Health Foundation's 2018 study found that 74% of people had felt so stressed that they have been overwhelmed or felt unable to cope in the past year. When these statistics were separated out it showed that the majority of young adults felt overwhelmed - or unable to cope - at times although only 30% of older people reported feeling like this.

Feeling overwhelmed negatively affected behaviour. Participants reported that they either ate unhealthily - or too much - started or increased their drinking, or started or increased their smoking.

The primary psychological effects, of those who reported feeling stressed, were depression and anxiety. Some of these participants had self-harmed and some had had suicidal thoughts and feelings. Stress also appeared to increase feelings of loneliness.

Regardless of the reasons for the stress – and there are indeed a great many; some of which we will visit later – the anxiety it often induces has been described as 'crippling.'

When we look at the definition of anxiety, it is defined thus:

Anxiety is a normal response to stress or danger and is often called the 'flight or fight' response. This process involves adrenalin being quickly pumped through the body enabling it to cope with whatever catastrophe may come its way. The problem arises when this response is out of proportion to the actual danger of the situation, or indeed is generated when there is no danger present.

The above definition separates 'healthy' anxiety, which is presented when there is real danger, from the anxiety which is out of all proportion to the event.

To some extent, anxiety can be generated in one person because they lack coping strategies or knowledge to deal with problems which arise. When anxiety is generated through lack of coping skills, we can learn coping strategies.

Additionally, we could employ, where possible, someone to deal with the situation which we find stressful. (I always have someone to sort out any laptop problems that I have, for example).

Alternatively, we could ask other people in organisations - whose job it is to specifically deal with the problems we face - for help.

Sometimes, this is not enough to deal with situations which make us feel anxious. Anxiety can have a genetic component and can appear without any apparent trigger. It cannot always be resolved satisfactorily by learning new coping strategies although they can help.

Anxiety does need treating. Even though anxiety is not physically painful, it impacts more on people's lives than many common, yet debilitating, physical illnesses.

A recent World Health Organisation study compared depression with angina, asthma, diabetes and concluded that the impact of depression on a person's functioning was 50% more serious than the impact of any of the physical conditions as described above. At present 40% of disability worldwide is due to depression and anxiety.

There is more than one anxiety disorder and it is common to suffer from more than one anxiety disorder at a time. Agoraphobia and Obsessive Compulsive Disorder are examples of anxiety states. Agoraphobia is likely to have resulted from panic attacks and OCD may occur as a result of Generalised Anxiety Disorder.

PANIC ATTACKS ----→ AGORAPHOBIA

GENERALISED ANXIETY DISORDER---→ OCD

When we look at the difference between panic and anxiety, we can see that panic is an intense feeling which can often involve feelings of doom, palpitations and pins and needles. Anxiety lacks such physical symptoms. It is a psychological condition which causes the person to avoid situations which would increase their anxiety.

PANIC = PHYSICAL SYMPTOMS

ANXIETY = PSYCHOLOGICAL SYMPTOMS

Continually avoiding such situations, impacts on their quality of life.

Most people with stress related disorders and anxiety generally know the underlying causes of their conditions causing the symptoms they have.

It is not unusual to hear people saying, 'The children are stressing me out' or 'I'm really anxious about the interview I have tomorrow.'

What they have difficulty with is finding a solution to their problem. When a solution seems out of reach then a reaction can occur which is out of all proportion to the event. This generally manifests itself in excessive eating, drinking or smoking.

Unhealthy eating, drinking and smoking do not have to be the answers to crippling anxiety there is a better way forward.

This book will look at what happens in the body when an anxiety state is manifested, and what you can do about it so that you can take control of it.

The methods shown in this book will work even if someone has had an anxiety state for many years and this, regardless of whether the cause is due to environmental influences or is genetic in nature.

The flight or fight response

What is the fight or flight response?

This response is also known as the acute stress response. It refers to the way that we act physically when we feel threatened, either physically or mentally. During this event, hormones are released which prepare your body to either fight the threat or run away, to safety, from it.

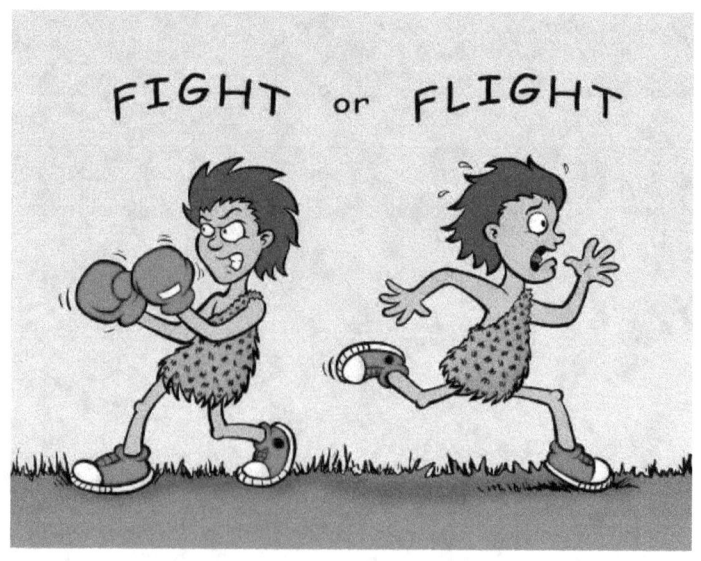

It is, in effect, a survival response to perceived danger in the environment. Whether we fight or flee is derived from the same underlying process. How we react will depend on our character traits and whether it would be foolish, or not, to face the danger head on.

The fight or flight response was not coined until the 1920's when it was described by an American Physiologist, Walter Cannon. He realised that there was a chain of reactions that occurred inside the body which enabled it to deal with perceived danger.

When acute stress occurs, the body's sympathetic nervous system is activated by a sudden release of hormones. The sympathetic nervous system brings about actions that aren't under our voluntary control. The adrenal glands, for example – which sit on top of the kidneys – are activated and trigger the release of cortisol.

Cortisol is an important hormone as it plays an important role in many bodily functions including the regulation of blood pressure, the functioning of the immune system and how the body uses glucose. For example, when you have an infectious disease the immune system is geared up to fight the infection by cortisol secretion. After extra cortisol is not required, your body goes back to a state of relaxation.

However, if cortisol production is continuous or prolonged as a result of stress, then high blood sugar, high blood pressure and a reduced ability to fight infections occurs. It also causes fat to be stored in the body.

Over time prolonged cortisol also impacts on the appearance of your skin.

When cortisol is raised, more of the circulating blood is diverted to the organs which will be needed to play a part in the fight or flight response. Thus, blood is diverted to the heart, brain, lungs and kidneys. Less is sent to the skin. People under prolonged stress often look tired, white and drained. Cortisol robs people of the pink tinge that people have on their cheeks when they are well.

Further, as cortisol and muscle tension go hand in hand, prolonged stress can also induce wrinkles. You may not be aware of what is going on inside your body but it can be seen on people's faces.

People under prolonged stress are generally (but not always)

- overweight with abdominal fat and rounded cheeks or
- have tight, drawn skin which is white and unhealthy looking

I have known people who are undergoing severe stress in their lives reporting that their doctors have told them to lose weight. Unfortunately, until the initial problem – stress – is dealt with, then it is highly unlikely that the patient could lose weight. Further, such comments only serve to increase the patient's stress levels even further.

Some key facts from the World Health Organisation[1] show that.

- Worldwide obesity has nearly tripled since 1975.
- In 2016, more than 1.9 billion adults, 18 years and older, were overweight. Of these over 650 million were obese.
- 39% of adults aged 18 years and over were overweight in 2016, and 13% were obese.
- Most of the world's population live in countries where overweight and obesity kills more people than underweight.
- 41 million children under the age of 5 were overweight or obese in 2016
- Over 340 million children and adolescents aged 5-19 were overweight or obese.
- Obesity is preventable

The pressures of living in the 21st century have no doubt fuelled the rise in obesity. Even

[1] https://www.who.int/news-room/fact-sheets/detail/obesity-and-overweight

though some experts will say that it is due to fast food and the availability of food, an individual that is not undergoing stressful events in their lives are unlikely to eat more than their body requires. All food, whatever source it comes from, is broken down into glucose, amino acids and fatty acids. The body then selects what it needs from these components to use as fuel, growth or repair. The rest is stored in fat cells. It matters not one bit whether the extra calories come from perceived 'healthy' food or not, they will still be stored as fat underneath your skin.

Fast food sometimes has less of the vitamins you might find in fresh food but this is not always the case. Some 'fresh' food, once cooked is unlikely to contain vitamin C since this is destroyed by heat.

Eating 'healthy' food when you don't particularly like it, is stressful in itself. The propensity to want to eat high carbohydrate food often stems from the stress response. Eating carbohydrates produces a ready source of energy ready to deal with the perceived threat.

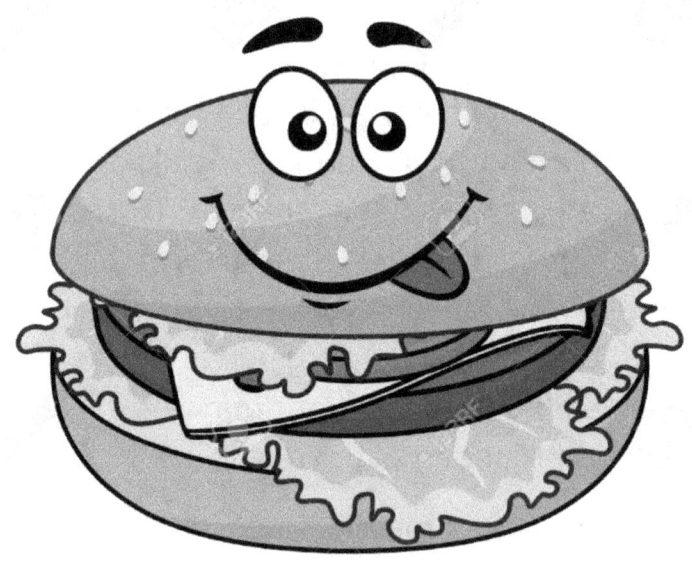

Fast food is not necessarily bad for you

We have learned that cortisol not only encourages the body to lay down fat in the long term but eating carbohydrate rich foods has a calming effect on the brain as well as provide instant energy to deal with the perceived threat. When stressful events arise, the individual is self-medicating, that is using food in order to calm themselves down. There is little point in going on a diet when the threatening circumstances – whether perceived or real - are still evident. This will just increase stress levels.

In a similar vein, nicotine – often used to alleviate anxiety - creates an immediate sense of relaxation but does not deal with the underlying issues causing the stress and feelings of anxiety.

Similarly, alcohol does have some sedating effects. It does depress the nervous system. However, it is easy to build a tolerance to alcohol so that it becomes less and less effective. The underlying reasons for the urge to drink alcohol have not been addressed.

Effects of Cortisol

Urge to pass urine/empty bowels – this is part of the stress response which makes sure that our bladder and bowels are empty before we start fighting.

Tremor and sweating - normally we sweat in response to external heat sources or physical activity. This is produced by eccrine glands. The sweat from stress is not a heat sweat and is produced by your apocrine glands. The tremor is also a result of the revved up responses going on in your body that are fuelled by cortisol.

Pins and needles – this is due to an active stress response. The cortisol diverts blood to vital organs. Those which aren't vital will constrict and tighten which can give rise to the feeling of pins and needles.

The psychological symptoms of anxiety are

- Agitation
- Tension
- Irritability
- A feeling of being detached
- Fear of losing control of the situation
- A feeling of impending doom

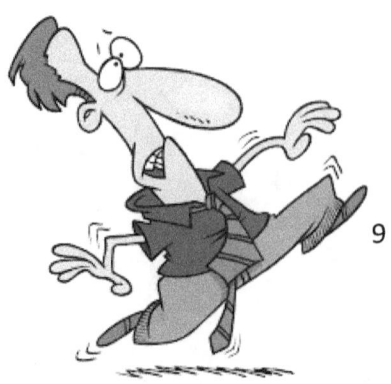

Anxiety causes agitation

External causes of stress

The pace of the 21st century and the rapid development in technology which is supposed to make our lives easier has had an unforeseen effect. While it may make some jobs easier to perform, this means that we can fit more of it in to our lives.

The knock on effect is that we are required to undertake more multi-tasking of complex events rather than the more linear and often 'therapeutic creative type tasks (joinery for example) which were undertaken more in the past.

The rise of the internet and everything which is related to it creates more noise, pressure and blue light.

Blue light is responsible for keeping us awake. It is emitted from TV screens, tablets, computer screens and similar. It prevents the synthesis of melatonin which is the hormone responsible for the sleep-wake cycle.

The lack of sleep which occurs when we are constantly exposed to the effects of the 21st century, have become so much a part of our lives that we no longer recognise how much it is negatively impacting on our lives. For young adults and children, they will never have lived in an era when this pollution did not exist. They cannot envisage what life was without all these gadgets. Stress and anxiety has become the 'normality' for them. It is not surprising that our children are becoming fatter.

Other causes of stress have been cited as:

- Health problems whether the individual's own or another member of the family. This was more prevalent the older a person got.
- Debt is also a stressor
- !2% of people reporting high levels of stress reported that this was due to having to respond to messages instantly.

- Body image
- Pressure to succeed
- Housing worries

The Naturally Anxious Person

Some people seem to be naturally anxious types. They are constantly on the go, can't sit still and worry about anything and everything.

Anxiety is a feeling of unease such as worry or fear. It can be mild or severe.

Some anxiety is normal. If we are going for a driving test, a college exam or meeting someone for the first time, then these can all cause anxiety which is perfectly normal.

When we are looking at **abnormal** anxiety it is the sort of anxiety which takes over the whole of people's lives.

Anxiety can be a symptom of other conditions such as

- PTSD
- Phobias
- Panic disorder
- Social anxiety disorder or social phobia

Generalised Anxiety Disorder (GAD) is a long term condition that causes people to worry about a wide range of situations and events rather than one particular focus. They never seem to be able to relax.

People with GAD can have both physical and mental symptoms which include:

- Sleeplessness
- Trouble concentrating
- Feeling worried
- Feeling restless
- Feeling dizzy

GAD can have a number of causes. These include

- An imbalance of chemicals in the brain such as

- Genes can play a part so if you have anxious parents then there is a good chance that it will be passed on. However, anxiety can have an environmental cause and simple be a learned response from others.
- Over activity in the areas of the brain that are involved in emotions and behaviour.
- Drug or alcohol misuse
- Having been abused or bullied as a child or a number of traumatic experiences at any time.
- Having a chronic illness

Sometimes no underlying cause can be found but GAD is found slightly more in women and in the age group from 35 -55 although it is not clear why.

Treatment for GAD

Treatment for GAD normally involves talking therapies such as CBT and/or medication such as selective serotonin reuptake inhibitors also known as SSRI's. These are antidepressants and work by increasing the level of a chemical in your brain called serotonin.

Serotonin is made from an amino acid called tryptophan which is found in carbohydrates. This is why people who are feeling stressed have a tendency to eat a high carbohydrate diet.

Antidepressants such as sertraline can be taken long term but a low dose will be started on first and increased gradually.

The difficulty with SSRI's is that they do not appear to work for a number of weeks and they can have quite a number of unwanted sided effects such as:

- Feeling or being sick
- Diarrhoea or constipation
- Loss of weight
- Indigestion
- Insomnia
- Excessive sweating

- Headaches
- Erectile dysfunction

If the SSRI's aren't effective. then a serotonin and noradrenaline reuptake inhibitor (SNRI's) may be prescribed. **This type of medicine increases the amount of serotonin and noradrenaline in your brain.**

The general function of noradrenaline is to get the brain and body ready for action. The amount of noradrenaline is at its lowest during sleep and at its highest during situations which involve the flight or fight response.

In the brain, noradrenaline increases arousal and alertness. It helps memory and helps focus attention. It can also cause anxiety and restlessness. This isn't helpful taking a medication which causes anxiety and restlessness for anxiety.

Further side effects of noradrenaline include an increase in heart rate and blood pressure which is not desirable. It also reduces blood flow to the gastro intestinal system and puts the brakes on voiding of the bladder. It can also cause constipation. So, just like SSRI's, SNRI's also have some nasty side effects. In fact, anxious people are likely to be made even more anxious by the side effects.

Sometimes, anticonvulsants, like Pregabalin – are prescribed. Pregabalin is well known for one of its side effects – that of huge weight gain. Most people can get very anxious when they start piling on massive amounts of weight.

On occasions, a benzodiazepine will be prescribed such as diazepam (Valium) but as these are addictive they are rarely prescribed for more than 2-4 weeks.

As the first two classes of medication can cause intense anxiety and agitation as some of their side effects then clearly they are better avoided if possible since we are trying to treat the anxiety not induce even more.

Pregabalin is an analogue of GABA. An analogue is something which is similar or comparative to another thing. Thus, pregabalin has been made to act like GABA. GABA is an inhibitory neurotransmitter with calming qualities.

Pregabalin has a structural resemblance to GABA but in spite of this, it does not have any activity in GABA's neuronal systems. In this respect, gabapentin – another popularly prescribed GABA analogue - is like pregabalin.

Pregabalin and gabapentin are used in seizure disorders and pain syndromes as well as generalised anxiety disorders.

Many people appear to feel calmer initially with pregabalin and gabapentin but after a short time often begin to experience sleeplessness, fatigue, weight gain and anxiety. These drugs, however do, however, appear to be good at treating neuropathic pain.

Weight gain isn't the only side effect of these GABA analogues either. When we look at some of the common symptoms – common symptoms occur in up to one in ten people - they include:

- Increased appetite
- Feeling confused or disorientated
- Less interest in sex and erectile dysfunction
- Feeling irritable
- Difficulty in concentrating
- Forgetting things
- Shaking
- Speaking difficulties feeling drunk
- Vertigo
- Problems with balance
- Constipation
- Feeling and being sick
- Having a bloated or swollen gut
- Swelling of the body, fingers and toes
- Muscle cramps, joint pains, back pain in arms and legs

which is really enough to make anyone feel anxious.

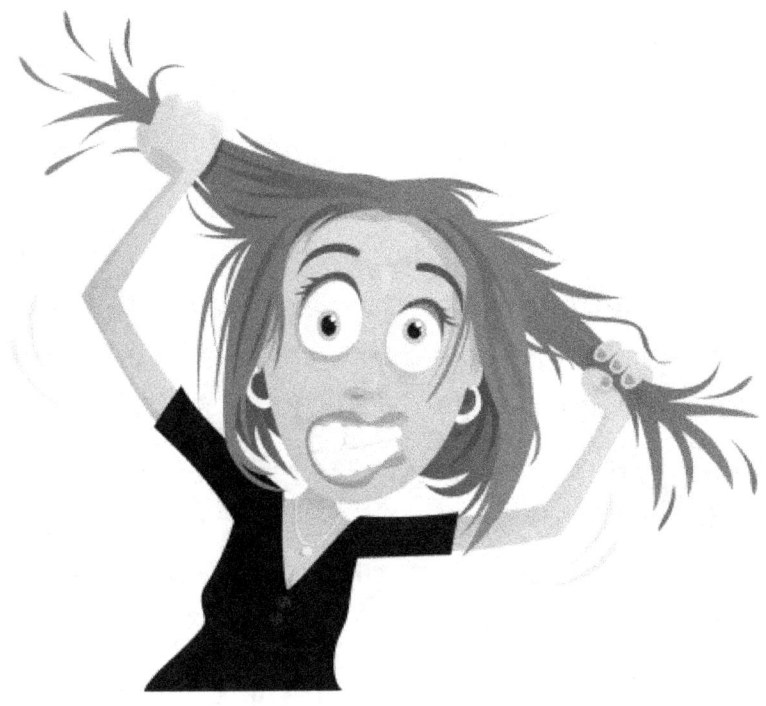

When you look at the medications with an anti-depressant effect then the main brain chemicals which they are hoping to increase are:

- Gamma amino butyric acid (GABA)
- Noradrenaline
- Serotonin

We have already looked at the way in which noradrenaline works so we will now look at the two calming neurotransmitters and see what they do.

When we have looked at them all in turn we will turn our attention to how we can increase these brain chemicals naturally so that we aren't reliant on prescription medication.

Serotonin is a chemical that has a wide variety of functions in the human body. It is sometimes called the happy chemical as it gives a feeling of wellbeing and happiness.

Serotonin is mainly found in the bowels, brain and blood platelets. It helps to constrict smooth muscle and it is also used to transmit messages between nerve cells.

It is a precursor for melatonin, which is the hormone involved in the sleep wake cycle. Clearly a lack of serotonin will impact on the ability to get a good night's sleep.

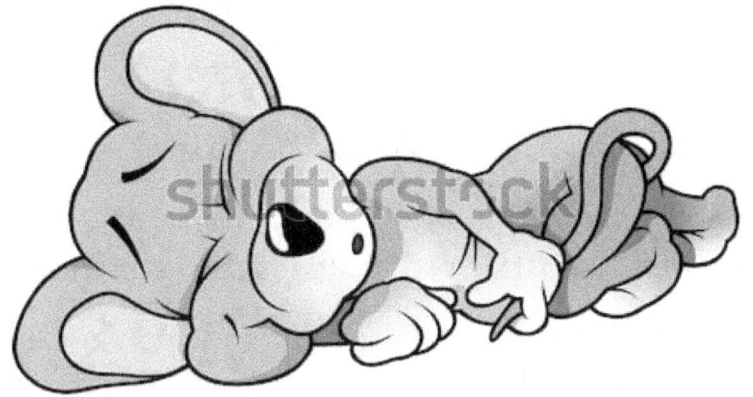

Serotonin helps you sleep

Further, it has a number of other roles which include:

- Regulating the appetite
- Improving mood
- Regulating motor, cognitive and autonomic functions
- Serotonin helps prevent the relaxed state of blood vessels which progress into a migraine, as well as treating nausea.
- It may also have a role in preventing obesity and Parkinson's disease

Body serotonin can be increased by getting plenty of daylight, exercise and a diet rich in complex carbohydrates which provides tryptophan which is a precursor to serotonin.

As serotonin cannot cross the blood-brain barrier, it must be produced inside the brain.

There is an indirect association between anxiety and increased gut motility. When people are anxious they generally increase their intake of carbohydrates which has a calming effect. The increase in carbohydrates results in the production of more serotonin which increases gut motility.

However, increasing levels of serotonin may result in an increase in osteoporosis.

A number of fairly recent studies have found that SSRI's may lower bone mineral density in those over the age of 65. However, those with depression – not taking SSRI's – are also at an increased risk of lower bone mineral density and hip fractures.

How this comes about is not exactly clear. Serotonin transporters have been found in osteoblasts[2], osteoclast[3] and osteocytes[4].

Animal studies have indicated that when there is disruption in the serotonin transporter genes then bone mineral density is significantly lower.

The evidence in humans is not as clear cut although Fluoxetine has been shown to decrease osteoblast formation and osteoclast differentiation in vitro.[5]

Nevertheless, it would be wise to take care of bone health by eating nutrients such as magnesium, boron, calcium and vitamin D and undertaking exercise to encourage bone building.

---

[2] Osteoblasts are responsible for new bone formation
[3] Osteoclasts are responsible for age bone resorption
[4] Osteocytes are bone cells
[5] Haney EM, Chan BK, Diem SJ, Ensrud KE, Cauley JA, Barrett-Connor E, Orwoll E, Bliziotes MM; for the Osteoporotic Fractures in Men Study Group. Association of low bone mineral density with selective serotonin reuptake inhibitor use by older men. Arch Intern Med. 2007: 167:1246-1251.

We all know that we feel better when the sun is shining. It lifts our spirits and makes us glad to be alive.

Both sunlight and darkness trigger the release of hormones in your brain. Indeed, in the winter months, many people suffer from a condition called Seasonal Affective Disorder and be affected badly by it.

They may suffer from depression, fatigue, irritability and eventually withdraw from society only to emerge from their 'hibernation' when spring arrives.

Exposure to sunlight triggers the release of hormones in the brain, especially serotonin. It imparts the 'feel good factor.'

At night time, however, serotonin production decreases and melatonin is synthesised instead. This hormone enables you to sleep.

Most people who work inside will not be exposed to an effective amount of light which would raise levels of serotonin. Some blue light is emitted from laptops and other screens but obviously this is not anywhere near as strong as sunlight.

Exercise is also able to raise serotonin levels. Studies have shown the clear association between exercise and mood which demonstrates antidepressant and anxiolytic effects.[6]

In fact, exercise has been recommended over antidepressants for treating depression as the risk benefit ratio is poor for use in patients with mild depression.

Further studies by Chaouloff[7] showed that exercise increased tryptophan in rat ventricles and more recent studies showed that exercise increases extracellular serotonin. [8]

---

[6] Salmon P. Effects of physical exercise on anxiety, depression, and sensitivity to stress: a unifying theory. *Clin Psychol Rev* 2001;21:33-61. [PubMed]

[7] . Chaouloff F, Elghozi JL, Guezennec Y, et al. Effects of conditioned running on plasma, liver and brain tryptophan and on brain 5-hydroxytryptamine metabolism of the rat. *Br J Pharmacol* 1985;86:33-41. [PMC free article] [PubMed]

A popular myth is that tryptophan from certain foods will cross the blood brain barrier to calm mood. This cannot happen as we have already seen.

All amino acids are transported into the brain via a transport system. This transport system is active towards all large neutral amino acids. Tryptophan is the least abundant and, in the competition between all the amino acids, tryptophan comes off worse.

The only way that tryptophan could cross the blood brain barrier via the transport system is if this amino acid was purified.

So saying this, alpha-lactalbumin contains more tryptophan than other amino acids and has been shown to improve mood.

In a similar vein, chickpeas have been shown to contain a lot of free form tryptophan.

---

[8] Wilson WM, Marsden CA. In vivo measurement of extracellular serotonin in the ventral hippocampus during treadmill running. *Behav Pharmacol* 1996;7:101-4. [PubMed]

Lentils also have a significant calming effect. If I serve them when I have guest around they generally nod off - either during the meal or shortly after.

Free form tryptophan is tryptophan which needs no digesting – it is readily available and it is quickly absorbed into the bloodstream to be used immediately for many metabolic functions. However, tryptophan needs niacin – vitamin B3 – in order for it to be converted to serotonin.

There have been some severe side effects with supplemental tryptophan so this is one amino acid which I recommend should always be obtained from food. This isn't as easy as it sounds but it can be done.

Why is it important that common antidepressants are not considered as the primary treatment for anxiety and related disorders? Well, a recent study [9] shows that

---

[9] https://www.medicalnewstoday.com/articles/319462.php?sr

they may pose a serious risk to health; they drastically raise the risk of mortality.

The study found that antidepressants.

'disrupt multiple adaptive, processes regulated by evolutionarily ancient biochemical, potentially increasing mortality.'

In other words, antidepressants disrupt lots of bodily functions which are normally regulated by a biochemical such as serotonin and can be fatal.

GABA

When we look at the effects of anxiety we find that it not only stems from disruptions in the brain but it can also cause them. Anxiety appears to be self-perpetuating resulting in a downward spiral from which there appears to be no escape.

Anxiety is not just very uncomfortable to live with but also is a risk factor for high blood pressure which is associated with heart disease, obesity and stroke.

Effects of anxiety

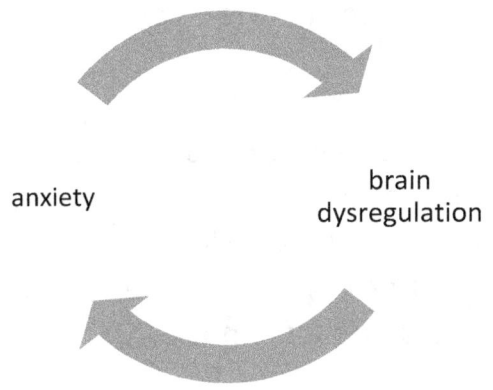

GABA is the primary inhibitory neurotransmitter that counterbalances, the rather excitable nature of glutamate – another neurotransmitter - from which it is converted.

Good sources of glutamate are:

- Mushrooms
- Cheese
- Milk
- Meat
- Fish
- Most vegetables

It is also made inside the body.

As we have already seen, a number of prescription drugs are GABA analogues – that is they try to fit into GABA receptors to produce the same effect. For some reason they do not work in the same way that GABA does.

One of GABA's main roles in the body is to reduce the activity of neurons in the brain and central nervous system. The induces a much calmer balanced mood, alleviates pain and helps you to sleep.

Some studies[10] show that GABA is 30% lower in those who suffer from insomnia than those who don't.

From my own personal experience of a lifetime of insomnia, once I started taking GABA I was able to sleep through the night and the irritability that the insomnia caused, also disappeared.

There are a number of natural supplements which help GABA achieve its function. These include:
- L theanine
- Hops
- valerian
- magnesium

GABA can be found in varieties of most common types of tea leaves which is why we naturally lean towards having a cuppa when we are feeling particularly stressed. It can also be found in fermented foods such as yogurt.

There are many other foods which either contain GABA or help increase its production in the body. These include:

---

[10] https://www.ncbi.nlm.nih.gov/pubmed/19014069

- whole grains
- soya
- lentils and beans
- nuts
- sunflower seed
- fish
- cocoa
- broccoli
- potatoes
- chlorella

GABA is also thought to play a role in gut motility. This is useful as most people who experience anxiety also report increased gut motility. GABA also helps to control inflammation.

Low levels of GABA result in
- stress
- anxiety
- depression
- inability to concentrate
- insomnia
- myalgia (muscle pain)

The jury is out as to whether GABA can effectively cross the blood brain barrier to alleviate these problems. Regardless of this, some studies have shown that GABA is effective in lowering anxiety. Slowed brain waves were seen within an hour of taking GABA. Further, it appeared that GABA helped enhance immunity in people who are undergoing emotional stress.

Magnesium, hops and valerian also bind to GABA receptors which induce the calming effect. They are GABA analogues just like gabapentin and pregabalin but without the negative side effects that these prescription medications have.

This ability to bind to GABA receptors also explains why magnesium is known as the calming mineral and is well known for alleviating pain. Unlike, GABA however, magnesium can have a loosening effect on the bowel whereas, as we have already discussed, GABA can have a constipating effect.

L- theanine works slightly differently to the above named natural GABA analogues. We learned that the main excitatory (stimulating) nerve messenger was glutamate from which, strangely the calming GABA was made from.

Glutamate works in ways which carry pain, it is involved in learning and memory and should it leak into the extracellular spaces in the brain it can cause brain injury. It is thought to be responsible for the damage found in diseases such as motor neuron disease.

L-theanine blocks some of the receptors for glutamate so that they can't exert their effects which include:

- sleeplessness
- anxiety
- pain

However, in addition to this, L-theanine also stimulates production of GABA thus adding to its tranquilising effects. It does not produce sleepiness or impair motor behaviour. In fact, it can actually help improve alertness a little.

Further, while GABA tends to lower *general* blood pressure, L-theanine will help lower the *spikes* in blood pressure which occur at times of intense stress and anxiety.

L-theanine dosage generally starts at 200mg twice daily although up to 800mg in divided doses of 200mg four times daily have been taken safely. Be guided by the instructions on the package which can be bought in most health food stores and online.

The only sources of l-theanine otherwise are green or black tea and some obscure bay bolote mushrooms.

The dosage of GABA is usually 100-200mg daily for sleep, stress and anxiety. GABA can be bought online or in most health food shops.

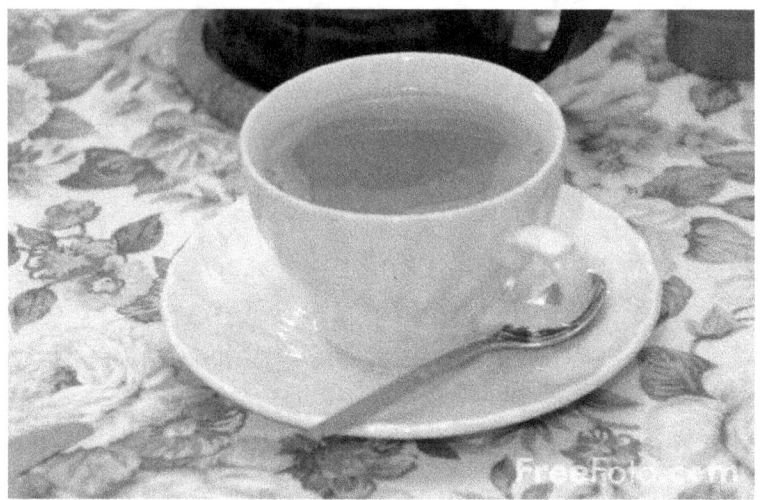
A cup of tea is a good source of L-theanine

GABA does not have many negative side effects and when they do occur they are generally only mild. These include:
- stomach upset
- reduced appetite
- constipation
- nausea
- burning throat
- drowsiness
- shortness of breath
- muscle weakness

As GABA is able to reduce appetite, it can be useful for treating people who overeat in response to stress.

Unlike prescribed medication for depression, stress and anxiety which is not effective for weeks, GABA and L theanine work in minutes if taken on an empty stomach. Further, there are no withdrawal symptoms should you wish to stop the above.

In contrast, prescribed antidepressants may have withdrawal effects for some significant time even if the user has been weaned off them gradually. Further, the initial negative side effects which are associated with this prescribed medication do not occur with L-theanine and GABA.

Noradrenaline – this is a naturally occurring hormone which can also act as a neurotransmitter - has been shown to play a role in depression, ADHD and low blood pressure.

Noradrenaline is released in the body in response to stress. It is called norepinephrine, alternatively.

Noradrenaline increases alertness and heart rate. It increases blood flow to muscles and releases glucose into the blood so that the body is primed for 'fight or flight.'

When noradrenaline acts as a neurotransmitter in the brain, it helps to increase arousal and motivation. It helps speed reaction time and ability to concentrate. However, low levels can result in the condition 'attention deficit hyperactivity disorder' which results in the individual having problems with attention and concentration. They find it difficult to focus because of the lack of noradrenaline.

Low levels of noradrenaline also result in depression and low blood pressure. The latter is because noradrenaline constricts blood vessels thus increasing the pressure required to push blood through vessels. Low levels of noradrenaline mean, of course, that the diameter of the blood vessels is relaxed so that less pressure is required to push blood through the blood vessels.

Low noradrenaline, as can be found in the condition ADHD, prevents people from solving problems. Planning and organisation are problematical, impulse control is poor and individuals with ADHD find it difficult to understand the perspective of others.

Most people have heard of Ritalin which helps ameliorate some of the effects of low noradrenaline and has the effect of helping an individual focus.

When we look at the effects of low noradrenaline these include:
- dry eyes and pin point pupils

- a decrease in calories burned which are needed to generate body heat in brown adipose tissue

- a decrease in fat burning in fat cells most people with ADHD are overweight)

- an increase in digestive activity

- dilation of blood vessels leading to low blood pressure

- in skeletal muscle a decrease in glucose uptake

- a decrease of glucose production

- In the kidneys lack of release of renin and loss of sodium

Most of this seems to sound like a miserable existence for the person with low noradrenaline levels.

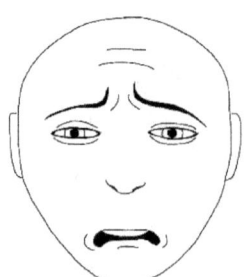

Low noradrenaline can make you depressed, stressed and anxious

At the beginning of this book we looked at some of the many negative side effects of antidepressants which help increase the availability of this neurotransmitter in the brain.

Their effect also includes increasing the availability of serotonin in the brain, regardless of whether levels of this neurotransmitter are low. Therefore, it appears prudent to look at natural sources of noradrenaline.

Before we consider this, noradrenaline is not the only neurotransmitter involved in the condition ADHD. Dopamine – a derivative of noradrenaline - is also involved in attention, focus and sustaining thought and alertness. Therefore, I shall examine natural sources of both of these chemicals.

Dopamine heightens energy, speeds up thought processes, increases assertiveness and aggression. People who find it difficult to assert themselves and have timid and fearful personalities are often short of dopamine.

Dopamine also promotes muscle coordination so a deficiency often results in an individual having dyspraxia which is often comorbid with ADHD.

Too much noradrenaline can result in anxiety and aggression, schizophrenia and psychosis.

People with lack of dopamine will often overeat in an attempt to supply themselves with the foods which will help increase dopamine and noradrenaline.

The effect of eating foods which help increase dopamine synthesis can be quite dramatic.
The protein foods that increase dopamine include red meat, fish, eggs, chicken, beans,

seeds, nuts, milk and tea.

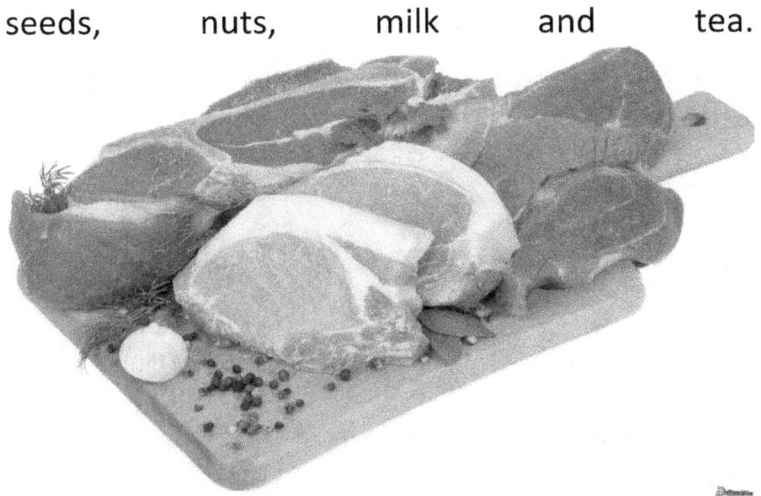

Meat is a great source of tyrosine

Once foods are eaten that are precursors of dopamine, the effect can be quite dramatic for it does not take long for amino acids to impact mood.

Ziggy Marley once said:

'The more red meat and blood we eat, the more bloodthirsty we get, the more violent we get. The more vegetarian food we eat; the more peace is taken into us.'

The ability to focus, assert and concentrate can happen very shortly after a meal which contains red meat and the other foods recently mentioned. Why do these foods work?

They contain an amino acid called tyrosine which your body needs to synthesise dopamine. This means that it is a building block of protein.

The body can make tyrosine from another amino acid called phenylalanine. Phenylalanine is often used as an adjunctive medicine alongside paracetamol and ibuprofen as it can enhance their pain relieving effects.

Tyrosine can be given to people who have learning and memory problems as it can increase alertness especially during stressful situations which are known to negatively affect memory, the ability to reason, attention and concentration.

Stress is known to decrease neurotransmitters. Tyrosine and phenylalanine are both used in the synthesis of:

- Thyroxine
- Melanin
- Norepinephrine
- Epinephrine

So the impact of stress on the human body should not be taken lightly.

A study showed that rats who were placed in cold conditions suffered stress and memory impairment but when tyrosine was administered to them, their ability to recall improved. In effect it reversed mental decline.

Humans studies have similar results.

Tyrosine also improves cognitive flexibility. Cognitive flexibility is the ability to multitask.

Tyrosine can also help with jet lag and enables people who are already sleep deprived stay alert.

Tyrosine has been said to help with depression because it can help with the production of neurotransmitters. Depression is said to be caused by an imbalance of neurotransmitters which is often caused by stressful situations.

Other studies do not support this. However, depression may be caused by a maladaptive response to environmental pressures such as relationship problems rather than poor eating habits which deprive the body of essential nutrients.

Let's face it, it is not difficult to eat a meal which is rich in tyrosine to see if it lifts mood. If it does and the individual also appears to have symptoms associated with ADHD, then it is fairly clear cut that changes in diet can help enormously with mood.

In fact, some studies support this. They have found that when depression is caused by dopamine deficiency then there is significant improvement when tyrosine supplements are given.

Tyrosine is considered to be a safe supplement. It can be supplemented at 150mg per kg of body weight daily for up to three months.

It is normally taken in doses of 500mg to 2000mg half an hour before intensive exercise.

Tyrosine should be used with caution if:
- Taking monoamine oxidase inhibitors as these can cause high blood pressure when certain foods such as cheese and beer are ingested.
- There is a problem with thyroid levels as tyrosine can affect them. It is a building block for thyroxine and it may synthesise too much
- L-dopa is a medication which is used for those with Parkinson's disease. The receptors for this are in the gut but tyrosine competes for these same receptors thereby interfering with the medications effects.

The importance of neurotransmitters for mental health

The role of neurotransmitters in treating anxiety, stress and depression is of vital importance in our understanding of mood disorders.

When we consider some of the pharmaceutically synthesised medications such as pregabalin which is often used to treat generalised anxiety disorder, it can be seen that although they are analogues and their structure is the same, they do not act in the same way as the natural analogues.

Natural analogues such as magnesium bind to GABA receptors and perform similar functions to GABA such as relieving pain and anxiety. This is why, wherever possible, we should eat to provide the nutrients we need for good mental health.

As we have already discovered, anxiety, stress and depression can be caused by poor diets.

If the building blocks of relevant brain chemicals are not available in the diet, then it is impossible to synthesise all the materials necessary for good brain health and emotional wellbeing. That is the bottom line.

Equally, there people who appear to have adequate diets who still suffer from stress, anxiety and depression. It may be that they have suffered particularly stressful events in their lives and their brain chemicals are depleted.

It may be that they are just inefficient at synthesising the necessary components needed for good mental health. We cannot rule the influence of genetics out.

If tweaks to the diet do not appear to alleviate depression or anxiety then I would recommend supplementation, to see if that works, since the results are often nothing short of miraculous if this is the problem.

This should also be a warning to those who eat a limited diet. It is often not a fast food diet that is the problem when treating mental health problems - a cheese burger, for example contains lots of tyrosine and serotonin – but a limited diet can be a problem if the full range of essential amino acids, in the right quantities, are not available when required.

It is not difficult to ingest more tryptophan than we require if we eat poultry all the time since poultry is high in tryptophan.

Eating foods high in tryptophan will give us the post prandial slump often seen after Christmas dinner has been eaten. This is when diners settle back into their comfy chairs for their 'forty winks.'

Red meat, while still containing all the essential amino acids, contains much more carnosine and carnitine than tryptophan. The post prandial slump is not a characteristic of the red meat dinner.

in addition to sufficient amino acids, adequate intakes of minerals and vitamins are needed to act as 'helper molecules' as they are involved in many biological processes that help to alleviate depression and anxiety.

Studies[11] have found, for example that zinc deficiency can lead to symptoms of depression, ADHD, difficulties with learning and memory, seizures, aggression and violence.

Another study[12] has shown that there is decreased zinc and increased copper in individuals with anxiety.

The three main sources of dietary copper are:
- Dark chocolate
- Organ meats

---

[11] https://www.psychologytoday.com/gb/blog/evolutionary-psychiatry/201309/zinc-antidepressant
[12] https://www.ncbi.nlm.nih.gov/pmc/articles/PMC3738454/

- Oysters

However, I do not think that the problem is an excess of copper in the diet for zinc deficiency is quite common throughout the world. It is this that I believe needs to be addressed.

People who are mainly on a plant based diet are at particular risk for zinc is found mainly in foods of animal origin. In addition, phytates in plants bind zinc so that it cannot be absorbed.

Zinc supplementation should be a serious consideration in those who eat little or no animal foods.

Low levels of B vitamins are known to cause depression, irritability and fatigue. Vitamins B6, B12 and folate deficiency are associated with anxiety and depression and are further, linked with a wide range of mental and physical health problems.

Vitamin B12 is only ever found in animal sources so supplementation is vital, in vegans and vegetarians, if a deficiency of this vitamin is not to occur.

Vitamin B12 also needs an acidic environment if it is to be detached from its protein source. The use of proton pump inhibitors, and other acid reducing medications, can also cause a deficiency of this essential vitamin.

The UK increasingly appears to be mass medicated with numerous prescription drugs whose side effects may not be immediately obvious but can impact mood and physical health.

The connection is not always made between new prescriptions and new symptoms. Why, people may ponder, should a drug to sort out my indigestion make me depressed? The thought is dismissed and put down to getting older or relationship problems.

Sadly, many relationship problems flounder because of mood disorders, due to poor diet, but the association is never made.

Niacin, vitamin B3 forms serotonin from tryptophan so something as simple as a vitamin B3 deficiency can cause mood disorders.

Numerous studies have shown that low levels of folic acid result in depression.

Good sources of folic acid are:

- Fortified breakfast cereals
- Spinach
- Chickpeas, pinto and lima beans
- Avocado
- Peas
- Brussels sprouts
- Green leafy vegetables

Niacin, folic acid and vitamin B12 (also known as cyanocobalamin) can be obtained very cheaply in supplement form as a vitamin B complex. Most UK supermarkets sell them for a couple of pounds.

The recommended amount of folic acid added to any supplement should not be more than

400mcg daily as it can hide a serious vitamin B12 deficiency.

Absorption of vitamins may become more problematical as you age even if you still have a varied diet. The quality of the food becomes more important especially as appetite appears to diminish as you age.

While many nutritionists say that you can obtain all the nutrients you need from your diet, I do not think that they have considered variables such as age. As such I do not frown on supplementation.

A nutritional sleeping tablet containing magnesium, calcium, tryptophan and vitamin B6 was marketed by Larkhall Laboratories. It was called *Somnamin.*

I have not been able to locate this sleeping aid but nevertheless, for those who like making their own health aids, this one would not be difficult to put together.

Glycine; anti-anxiolytic

Glycine is a star when it comes to a naturally occurring amino acid that reduces anxiety, pain and insomnia all in one go.

Glycine is a non-essential amino acid. This means that the body can synthesise it from other substances. It is not essential that we take it in through dietary means.

That's the hype anyway. Of course, we have to eat the foods that provide the building blocks of glycine so that it can be synthesised in the body and that doesn't always happen. Then, of course, there is that matter of aging when what our bodies did so well when we were younger, doesn't happen quite as efficiently.

It seems much simpler to eat foods containing glycine so we know that when digestion has broken our meal down, there will be the amino acid glycine, in its component part. However, there is a problem.

Nowadays, we eat little glycine in our diet. Glycine is found in the parts of the animal that we tend to throw away like the bones and skin. It is also found in organ meats that have fallen out of favour in our diets. It is found in the skin and heads of fish and in oxtail - both of which can make wonderful stock if only we had the time and the know-how. The truth is that we are losing the skills that used to be part and parcel of family medicine.

I do not know of anyone – apart from myself - who makes their own bone broth or soup from fish heads. Even liver and kidney have fallen out of favour in regular diets.

Glycine is the ultimate natural tranquiliser that we have eliminated from our diets since the immediate post war years. It was eaten regularly because nothing was wasted. The saying, 'Waste not, want not,' was on everyone's lips.

It is no wonder, that, wherever you look nowadays, there are angry, stressed people who are 'living on their nerves' and unable to sleep. Our diets contain far more red meat now and the end product of this diet is the stress hormone.

Our diets have become unbalanced and we have lost the skills that we needed to tweak diets to an expected result.

When glycine helps us to relax, to sleep, to reduce anxiety and pain, it is madness not to harness the power it has.

Further, unlike prescription antidepressants, glycine will begin to work within thirty minutes of it being taken in food. It will not cause a temporary disturbance of brain chemicals nor initial and worsening symptoms in the way that prescription medications do.

One of the best items that you can buy if you are serious about improving your mental health is a slow cooker to throw bones or a chicken carcase or fish heads into (take out the gills as they are bitter). In other words, get into the habit of making good stock.

Make it regularly; always have some in the fridge or freezer to use in soups, stews or risottos. It is delicious and the best medicine you can buy for stress and anxiety.

As an added bonus it is good for connective tissue, helps repair skin and soothes the pain of arthritis.

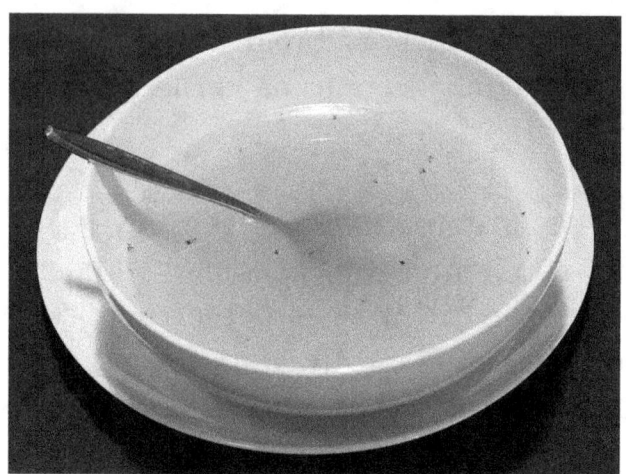

Bone broth has wonderfully soothing properties

To make bone broth

Take bones, skin or fish heads - depending on the type of stock that you want to make – throw them into the slow cooker with a little lemon juice and water to cover.

Cook on low for 6-7 hours (or overnight)

Drain stock into a container. Discard the bones, skin or fish heads. Let the stock cool. Pack for use in soups, risottos later.

Store for up to three months in the freezer and for up to three days in the refrigerator.

The addition of cooked lentils, if making a soup or stew with the stock, will increase the tranquilising effect. This is because lentils contain good amounts of tryptophan.

A mug of lentil soup made with bone stock - and drunk before bedtime - is guaranteed to ensure a good night's sleep.

Lentil Soup

Sweat lentils and onion in a small amount of butter on a low heat for a couple of minutes. Add stock to cover and simmer, stirring all the while. Keep adding stock as needed until the lentils have simmered in the stock for 25 minutes.

Add black pepper and more stock until desired consistency is reached. Blend. Add a little milk, if desired and thicken with a little cornflour, dissolved in water, if you require a thicker soup.

Other seasonings and vegetables can be added to the basic soup, to taste.

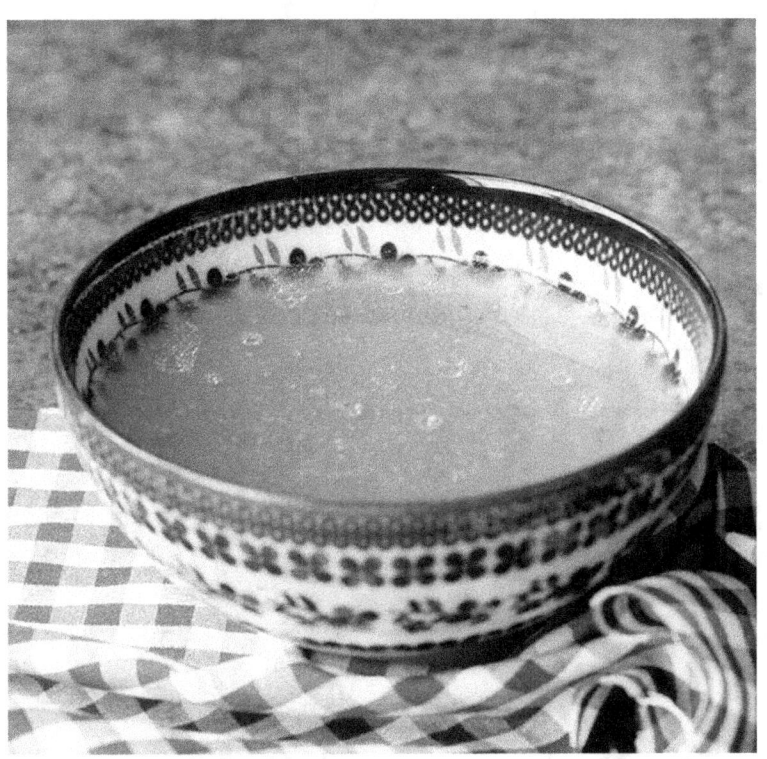

13   Bone broth relieves anxiety, depression, pain and insomnia

---

13

https://www.google.com/search?q=bone+broth&rlz=1C1GCEA_en GB828GB828&source=lnms&tbm=isch&sa=X&ved=0ahUKEwi30pL1 gpnhAhXaShUIHXOtC7MQ_AUIDygC&biw=1093&bih=500#imgrc= MVG0UjutK_6UUM:

If you do not have time to make bone broth or do not like cooking, then glycine can be obtained online quite easily.

It comes in crystalline form and tastes slightly sweet so it can be used to sprinkle over cereals or stirred into a hot beverage. You don't need more than a teaspoonful daily.

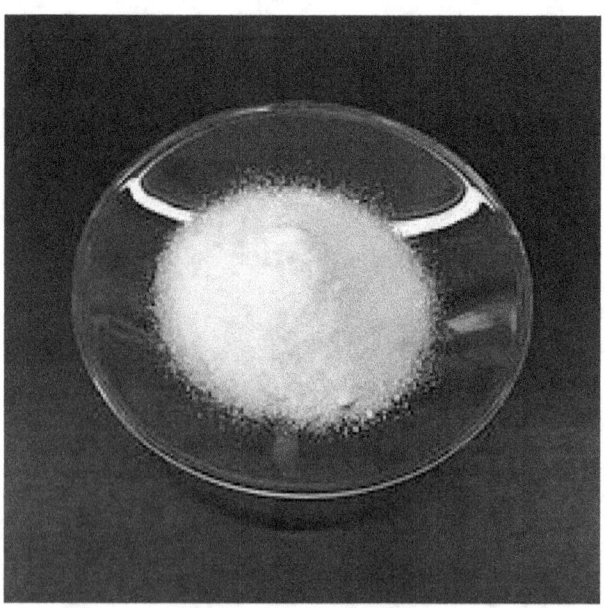

Glycine comes in granular form and tastes slightly sweet.

Nowadays, some children's medication is made into 'gummy bears.' The great thing about glycine that it can be bought in most shops selling **gelatine** sweets such as wine gums. Glycine accounts for 22% of the composition of gelatine. Vegan brands will not contain gelatine.

Many years ago, before I knew of this characteristic, I found that eating wine gums appeared to reduce any pain that I had within less than thirty minutes. To this end I always kept a bag of wine gums in the house.

It was no surprise to me on further investigation that the main amino acid was glycine and that it had analgesic properties.

Phenylalanine

We have touched upon phenylalanine and how it is needed to make tyrosine and subsequently makes dopamine which helps lift depression. Dopamine is involved with feelings of pleasure in the brain so its synthesis is vitally important to our mental well-being.

In addition, phenylalanine is known to help with pain, the stress response and some skin disorders.

Phenylalanine is an essential amino acid which means that your body cannot make enough for its needs and must be obtained from the diet.

Fortunately, this amino acid is found in a wide variety of foods and it is unlikely an individual would be deficient in it unless their diet was very poor or they had absorption problems.

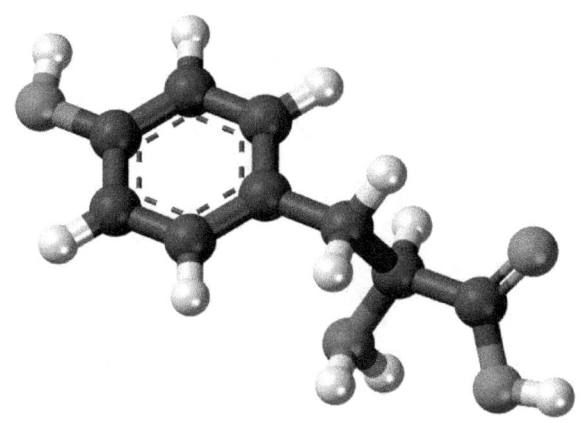

Phenylalanine is an essential amino acid

There is a genetic condition called phenylketonuria which some individuals have. In this, an error of metabolism means that the metabolism of phenylalanine is severely reduced.

This can lead to seizures, mental retardation and mental health problems. A diet low in phenylalanine needs to be followed if these symptoms of this condition are to be avoided.

However, for those who feel that a diet deficient in phenylalanine may be partially responsible for mood disorders then the foods which are highest in this amino acid are:

- Milk
- Eggs
- Cheese
- Chicken
- Beef
- Pork
- Fish
- Nuts
- beans

As you can see there are plentiful supplies of phenylalanine in both animal and plant dietary sources.

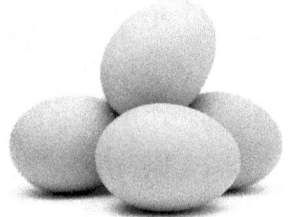

Eggs are a good source of phenylalanine

Low Potassium and Magnesium Levels

I don't see many books on nutrition making the association between low potassium levels and I believe that this is a serious omission.

I have already called to account the practise of mass medicating individuals with common prescription drugs as though they were harmless and would only address the symptom that the patient went to see the doctor for in the first place.

When I first started looking after elderly, I did not know of one that wasn't on a diuretic of some sort. It seemed to be standard practise to give anyone over the age of 55 years one.

In years before that, if people had swollen ankles they were encouraged to put their feet up for an hour in the afternoon to encourage the fluid to drain. A wedge of wood raised the bottom of the bed to assist this process overnight. Patients were advised to drink more fluid.

This may initially appear to be counter-productive to treating oedema but by increasing fluids, excess sodium is diluted and passed out of the body in urine. This was not so severe that it had a detrimental effect like the non-potassium sparing diuretics like Furosemide.

My cousin was on another diuretic called Indapomide. If you read the leaflet it clearly stated as one of the side effects, dehydration.

If you are dehydrated your natural response is to drink more so the whole action is pointless and deprives you of important micronutrients.

Potassium supplements are not recommended. Potassium is one of those trace minerals where you can easily get too much or too little off since the safe range is quite narrow.

Good sources of potassium are bananas and tomatoes – fresh, canned or juiced – potatoes, most fruits, cooked spinach, peas and mushrooms but this is not a definitive list by any means.

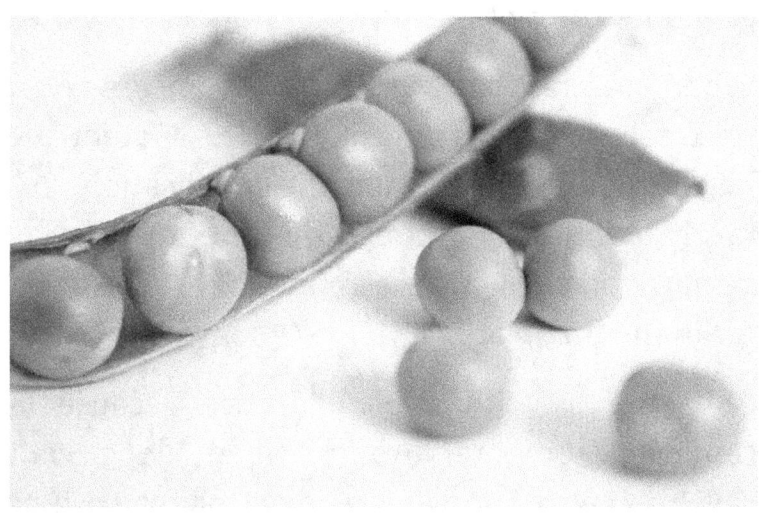

Peas are a good source of potassium

Nowadays, no-one has time to put their feet up or make meals containing less salt than the ready- made meals that most people seem to eat nowadays.

Anyway, most GP's do not readily give out advice on nutritional strategies. It is not a subject that they go into any great depth when in medical school and limited time face to face with patients means that it is often easier to give out prescriptions.

When prescriptions are given out they are given to treat specific symptoms. The potentially negative side effects of the medication are rarely mentioned although the side effects may be far worse than the ailment they were given for in the first place.

And so it is with many diuretics because in removing temporary excess fluid along with salt, they also remove vital electrolytes such as potassium and magnesium from the body.

Some of the more immediate side effects of low potassium are constipation, brain fog, depression, fatigue, confusion and hallucinations.

Longer term low potassium (hypokalaemia) can cause the breakdown of muscle tissue - including the tissue of the heart - and redistribute fat so that it builds up as visceral fat. Those people who are apple shaped tend to have a build-up of visceral fat which pumps out inflammatory chemicals which also can affect mood.

Magnesium is also flushed out of your system when you take non potassium sparing diuretics.

Magnesium is required for over 300 actions in the body and a deficiency has a major impact on both physical and mental health.

Fairly recent research has found that about three quarters of the world population are not having enough magnesium in their diet. That's a lot of people who cannot be living their life to the full.

The list of mood disorders due to hypomagnesia is a long one. It includes:

- lack of feeling and emotion
- numbness related to apathy
- increased risk of depression
- in severe cases, coma
- anxiety

Magnesium achieves its calming effect by blocking the receptor of a substance known as NMDA. NMDA is excitatory in action promoting pain signals and alertness, among other actions.

Magnesium inhibits NMDA from attaching to the cell and acts as the ligand

A ligand is simply something that attaches to a cell causing something to happen when it does so.

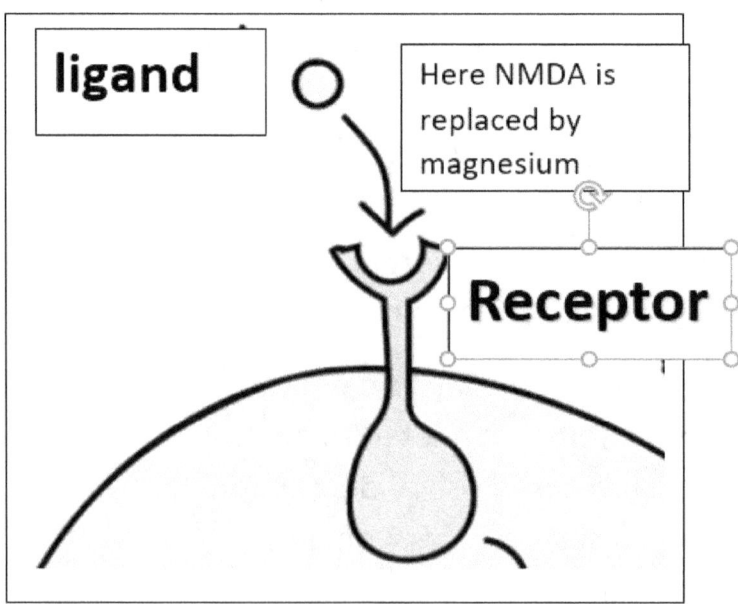

Simple diagram of ligand and receptor showing magnesium replacing NMDA

I have heard of many sorry souls say that they feel numb and have lost the ability to feel.

Magnesium is depleted very rapidly when and individual is going through stressful events. Given that they are, in all probability, already magnesium deficient then the outlook is not promising.

Magnesium deficiency is not easy to test for. Little of it ends up in the circulatory system. Most of it is inside cells and this makes it harder to test for.

Magnesium does not take long to exert and effect on mood – certainly not as long as some of the prescription drugs take that make you feel worse before they make you feel better - and it comes without side effects if taken in doses of 400mg daily for adults.

For the initial couple of days, it will not harm to take double that dose just to help restore magnesium equilibrium. Any excess will be excreted by the kidneys so the only contraindication for this nutrient is if you have poorly functioning kidneys.

I do wish that magnesium was recommended by GP's more often when a patient comes in with a mental health problem. It costs very little to buy over the counter. However, I suspect that if the GP is aware of magnesium's benefits for mental health there is also an awareness that such a simple remedy is hardly likely to make profit for pharmaceutical companies.

It disturbs me that simple treatments that can make such a dramatic impact on the quality of life for individuals is denied them either through deliberate withholding of this information or ignorance on the health professionals part.

People with mental health problems have the potential to be very vulnerable and deserve better treatment than they appear to be getting from country wide services.

At the very least, mental health charities should be looking into the possibility that lack of nutrients especially magnesium may be the cause of emotional numbness especially if it is concomitant with apathy and depression.

There are plenty of good sources of magnesium so a varied diet should provide all you require. Of course, there are groups that may be susceptible to hypomagnesia and these include:

- faddy eaters
- the elderly
- those with absorption problems
- the homeless and those who are unable to obtain a good mixed diet for whatever reason
- those who self-neglect
- those on calorie reducing diets

This is not by any means a definitive list. I am sure that you can add your own.

Good sources of magnesium include:

- nuts of all kind
- spinach
- cereals

- soy milk
- beans
- dark chocolate
- whole wheat bread
- avocado
- yogurt
- banana
- oatmeal
- cocoa
- milk
- beef
- broccoli
- vegetables – small amounts

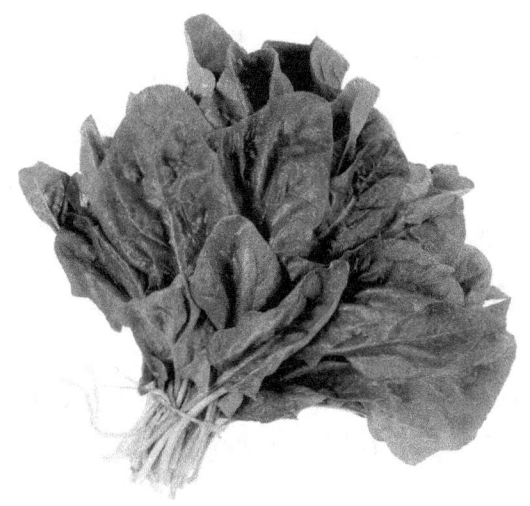

Spinach contains good amounts of magnesium

Altered pH; Altered mental state

I hardly ever see reference to an altered pH as being responsible for mental health problems yet there is enough research on it to take this aspect seriously.

Metabolic acidosis is implicated in many disease states yet very few people have heard of it or how it may impact health.

Metabolic acidosis develops when too much acid is produced in the body or if the kidneys and lungs are unable to remove enough acid from the body. The pH of the blood should be around 7.4 and anything lower is referred to as acidosis whilst anything higher is referred to as alkalosis.

Metabolic acidosis can cause serious health issues and may be life threatening.

The excess acid may occur due to lactic acid (produced during exercise) or ketoacids.

There are three main ways that ketoacidosis can come about. These are through:

- Alcohol
- Being in a diabetic state
- Starvation

I shall look at these in more detail later.

It may occur due to the loss of bicarbonate which may occur for a number of reasons including the ageing process.

It may occur due to the reduced ability of the kidneys and lungs to excrete excess acid. Therefore, people with lung conditions such as asthma or COPD, for example, are at particular risk.

Depression is comorbid with lung conditions and it is helpful to know why.

It is also prevalent in conditions such as diabetes and, as these conditions affect a large part of the population it is helpful to understand why and what we can do to address this.

As acidosis can start in the lungs or the kidneys then we can divide them into two separate categories. Each of them has their own specific symptoms and it is easier to compare them if they are tabulated for convenience.

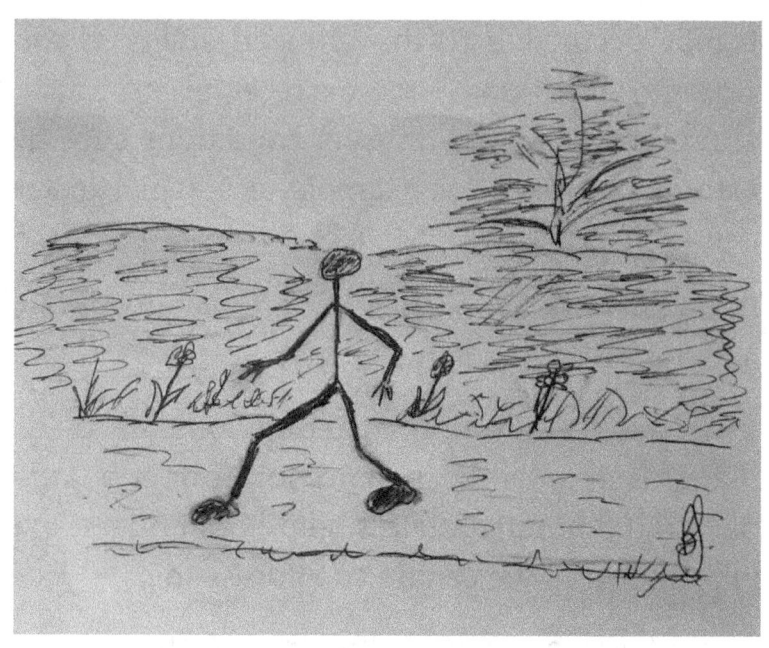

Excessive exercise can induce ketoacidosis

Table showing the symptoms of respiratory and metabolic acidosis

Respiratory acidosis	Metabolic acidosis
Drowsiness	fatigue
Easy fatigue	Confusion or severe anxiety due to hypoxia
Shortness of breath	Rapid shallow breathing
Headache	headache
sleepiness	Sleepiness coma lethargy decreased visual acuity
confusion	Loss of appetite nausea vomiting abdominal pain altered appetite weight gain
	Diabetic acidosis (breath smells fruity) and Kussmaul respirations (deep rapid breathing associated with diabetic ketoacidosis)
	jaundice
	Tachycardia (increased heart rate)

	abnormal heart rhythms (eg ventricular tachycardia) and low blood pressure due to decreased response to epinephrine
	Joint and bone pain muscle weakness

I have already touched on the point that ketoacidosis can occur due to alcohol, a diabetic state and/or starvation. As diabetes - and the potential to starve oneself – is tied in with metabolic syndrome, then it would be wise to look at this condition a little further.

Diabetic ketoacidosis is a serious complication of diabetes. It develops when your body cannot produce enough insulin and ketones are produced as a source of energy from the breakdown of fat.

The signs of diabetic ketoacidosis are that blood sugar levels will be high (hyperglycaemia) as will ketones.

There are testing kits for both.

The symptoms of this condition include:

- More frequent urination
- Thirst
- Pear drop breath
- Drowsiness
- Stomach pain
- Feeling or being sick
- Confusion
- Passing out
- Deep fast breathing

Starvation ketosis occurs when the glycogen stores in the liver are exhausted and energy must be obtained from the breakdown of fat stores.

This may start between 15-24 hours of fasting or but gathers pace the longer the period of starvation.

Clearly, while we may want the weight loss, we do not want a state of acidosis with all the signs and symptoms that go with that.

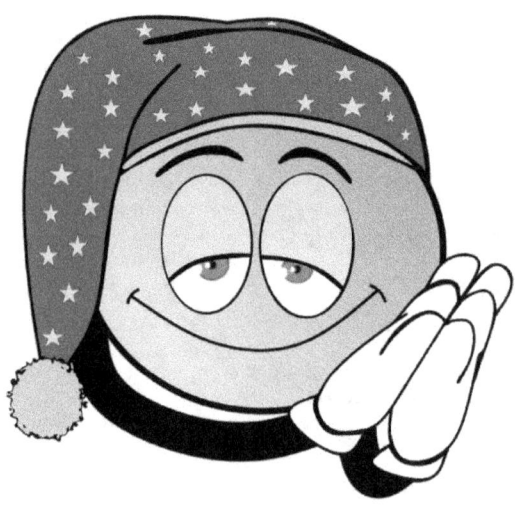

Metabolic acidosis can make you feel very sleepy

Dr Mark Sircus, in his book Sodium Bicarbonate Nature's Unique First Aid Remedy cites the dosage of sodium bicarbonate as provided by Arm and Hammer for oral use for metabolic acidosis

This is:

- Add half a teaspoon of bicarbonate of soda to half a glass of water and take every two hours

Do not take more than three half teaspoons if you are over 60 years of age.

Do not use this maximum dosage for more than two weeks.

As many of the problems that occur with dieting – such as headache and loss of energy – are due to the body being in a state of ketoacidosis then it makes sense to add one teaspoon of bicarbonate of soda to a glass of water and take this at any point during the day. If you prefer you can sip it over the day.

You may not lose huge amounts of noticeable weight during this time because the sodium can cause slight oedema. However, if you take plenty of foods containing potassium and magnesium this should counteract this tendency.

At the end of two weeks it is preferable if you reduce the sodium bicarbonate but there is always the option of increasing it if the symptoms of ketoacidosis occur.

The best way to test whether the body is in an acid state or not is through the use of saliva or urine tests.

To test for saliva, wait until 2 hours after eating then fill the mouth with saliva and test with litmus. It should go blue. A healthy alkaline state should be between 7.1 and 7.5.

Anything less than 7.1 places you in an acidic state and needs to be remedied by the addition of some bicarbonate of soda in water as outlined above.

You can test as many times as you like for the pH.

With urine tests the expectation is that the pH range will be between 6.5 to 7.5 on the urinalysis strips. If the test reveals that the pH is lower, then you follow the regime mentioned above until a state of health returns.

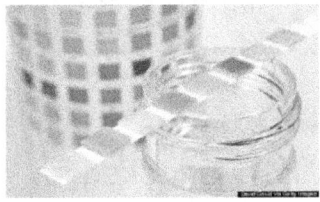

Urinalysis is a straightforward process

All you need to do is dip the stick into fresh urine and read it off the chart you will find wrapped around the container.

Clearly, bicarbonate of soda is useful in preventing the lethargy and headachy type symptoms that often accompany the initial stages of a calorie controlled diet or diets which rely heavily on protein or fat and thus produce a state of acidosis.

However, there are no studies that have found that taking sodium bicarbonate will directly help with weight loss but as one of an arsenal of weapons it has considerable value.

It is cheap, easily obtainable in any supermarket and it deserves a place in the overall strategic plan to recover from metabolic syndrome.

Its only drawback is that such simplicity may mean that it is overlooked as an adjunctive treatment for a complex condition that affects approximately one third of the population.

By now, my hope is that I have persuaded you to understand that many of the mental health problems that we currently see in society are not due to weak individuals with poor coping strategies but are the result of a deficiency of some nutrient or other.

Many mental health problems appear in the teen years when there is greater control over what is eaten and what is eaten may be limited so that the culturally accepted stick thin figure can be maintained.

The downside to this is that as anxiety and depression set in and prescription medicine is offered, then the main side effects are intolerable weight gain, brain fog and confusion.

The demands of university may require a diet that leans heavily towards foods containing magnesium if the stresses that inevitably arise with studying are managed well.

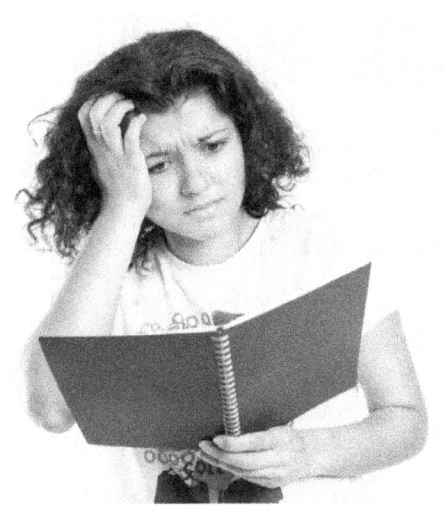

Studying can be stressful and require a varied diet in order to cope with the stress.

There are other particular times in an individual's life which make them susceptible to depression and anxiety.

The arrival of a new baby is one such time. Post-natal depression may set in but it is not always the case that it occurs because of the new mother's anxiety about being a parent. The pregnancy and birth are themselves stressful events and require nutrients like magnesium to help cope with them. Nevertheless, although I have heard pregnant mothers told to be careful of their iron levels - and sometimes of their vitamin D levels - I have never heard of them being informed they should be mindful of their magnesium levels.

What I would like to see is a nutritionist who has a special interest in mental health disorders, attached to every health care practice. Before the doctor even hands out a prescription for any mood disorder, the patient should be referred to this nutritionist for a thorough appraisal of their diet. This should also form the first of many meetings.

If necessary, patients could be referred to classes where they could learn useful cookery skills that they may not have.

We do this at the moment with people who are deemed overweight by sending them to free gym classes or slimming classes, so it seems reasonable to teach skills to those to whom it may ultimately improve mental health for.

Doctors know that poor nutrition and a depletion of brain chemicals are responsible for mental health problems. They know that food can provide those missing chemicals but it is so much easier to provide pills than spend a little time searching for the underlying reason.

In many ways this makes the patient more dependent on a health system which is already failing due to lack of funding. They simply never learn what is the underlying cause and how to address it through bespoke nutrition. They will always be dependent on the appointment system, a face to face consultation before being handed a prescription.

I know of many fine intelligent people who are the salt of the earth but when I find they are on medication – and I know them well - I ask them why they were put on it and what are the side effects and alternatives.

On every occasion, none of them have been able to answer any of those questions yet some have been on prescription medicine for over a decade without any follow up in that time.

Some other causes of depression are:

- Statins
- Low fat diets

My fervent hope is that this book will reach some people and help them begin to make that important step to changing their lives for the better.

The B vitamins

I do not think that any book written on the subject of stress, anxiety and depression is complete without looking at the contribution that the group of vitamins known as the B complex have to mental health. I have known miraculous recovery in days of people who have followed the thiamine regime that I will add at the end of this chapter. In many respects I have saved the best until nearly last.

When I mention miraculous recovery, I do not use these words lightly. Within hours to days, those with suicidal tendencies are not suicidal anymore. Those with depression no longer need to take anti-depressants although it would be true to say that most of the latter do not work anyway. Those who are prone to aggression, apathy, brain fog, lack of clarity when speaking who are anti-social, stressed, suffer from intolerable anxiety, agoraphobia or indeed, any other phobia, suddenly find that all this begins to lift and fairly rapidly, too.

Although the B vitamins work together synergistically, there are one or two that I am going to pick out to highlight in greater depth. Most people have heard of vitamin B12. Indeed, many people take vitamin B12 - it appears to be quite fashionable at the moment – without really understanding most of its vital functions but they do take it having some subconscious knowledge that it may be beneficial to do so.

However, If I was to ask people what thiamine does – and I do quite often- people do not know of the miraculous powers of this vitamin when given in therapeutic doses. That is, in far higher doses than the recommended daily intake of 1.4mg approximately which is a pittance given the deficiency of thiamine which is rife in society at the moment.

Thiamine deficiency is the great mimicker of hundreds of other diseases. It has been mooted – and I tend to agree with this position – that thiamine is the root cause of most of the neurodegenerative disorders that there are.

How does thiamine function?

In every cell there are tiny organs (organelles) called mitochondria. Mitochondria are the powerhouses of the cell and take fuel (carbohydrates for example) and oxygen to form energy. However, this cannot take place without thiamine as a cofactor. A cofactor is a non- protein substance such as a vitamin which works with other substance to cause something to happen. Thiamine actually works like a spark plug igniting the fuel and oxygen to produce energy.

Mitochondria are found in every cell in the body. If there is a thiamine deficiency, then it could impact any part of the body. However, there are well-recognised systems which appear to be particularly affected and these are the cardiovascular system, the nervous system and the gastrointestinal system.

A deficiency of thiamine is implicated in mood disorders, Alzheimer's disease, Parkinson's disease, motor neuron disease, vascular dementia, seizure disorders, stroke. Central nervous system disorders caused by a thiamine deficiency are known as dry beriberi. As it progresses it may result in Wernicke's encephalopathy and if it progresses further then it results in Korsakoff's syndrome. While the encephalopathy is generally associated with excessive alcohol intake and the Korsakoff's syndrome definitely is, there are still many, many cases that occur due to malnutrition, poor absorption (even with a good diet) and the inclusion of foods which inhibit or destroy thiamine such as:

Tea, coffee, raw fish (sushi and shellfish) alcohol, high carbohydrate diets.

Then there is the necessity of making sure that there is enough magnesium in your diet because magnesium is an activator of thiamine. Without magnesium, thiamine will not be able to function as it should.

Medications such as diuretics flush away thiamine and magnesium so that it cannot be utilised by the body.

Metformin, a common diabetic medicine can cause a deficiency of thiamine within days. It is also a risk factor for lactic acidosis which is another condition which can make you feel very unwell indeed.

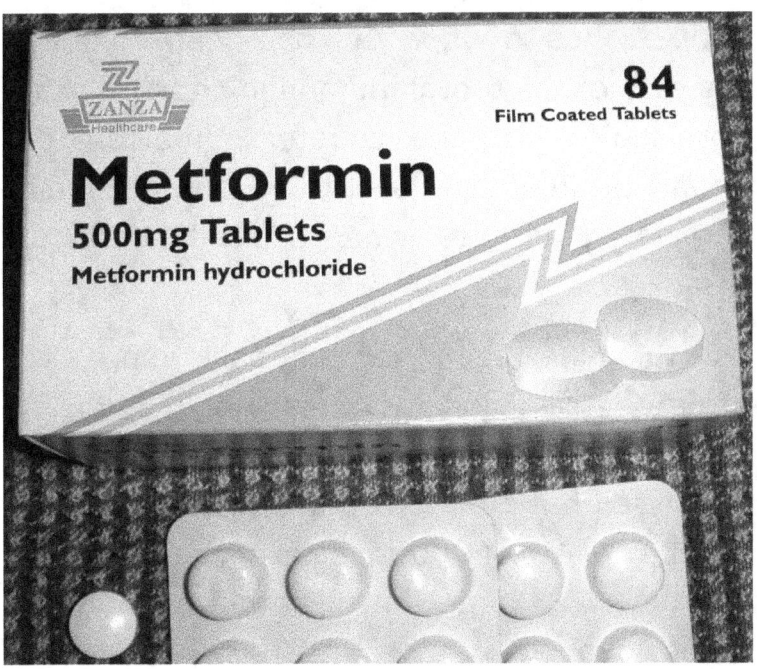

Metformin can reduce levels of thiamine very quickly causing mood disorders in the process.

The proton pump inhibitors block the absorption of magnesium and thiamine among other vital nutrients. These are medications which are prescribed far too easily without any consideration of the wide reaching impact on people's health when this has been done. In the case of the proton pump inhibitors they are obtainable over the counter. Unfortunately, people often equate 'over the counter' as being completely harmless when this is far from the case.

The thiamine regime can roll back depression, anxiety, stress and insomnia within hours. I know because not only have I experienced this for myself but hundreds of people have written to me of their positive experiences of thiamine. Some are nothing short of miraculous.

The thiamine regime

Take 300mg of thiamine in 3 divided doses throughout the day along with

300mg of magnesium and

A good vitamin B complex

If you do not feel any difference after one week (this would be very unusual) then increase to 600mg for one week. Increase in 300mg doses weekly until you have reached 900mg. Please eat high magnesium foods during the day as well as taking the magnesium supplement and B complex.

If there is absolutely no improvement when you have reached 900 mg then you need to start rolling back 300mg weekly until you reach 100mg where, if you so wish, you can continue on this dosage.

Now and again it is good to take a break from any supplement so a break of six weeks every 3 months or so should be considered.

Good food sources of thiamine are:

Malt and malted milk products, yeast extract, whole meal and fortified foods, nuts, liver and organ meats. Pork muscle meat has probably the highest amount.

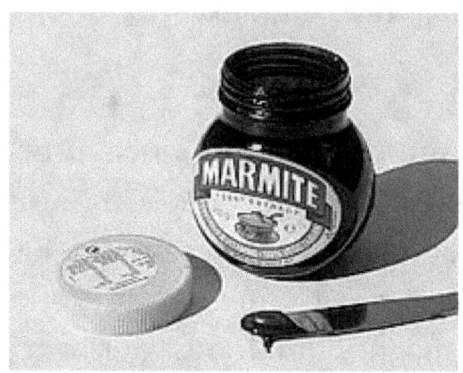

Yeast extract is a good source of thiamine and B vitamins in general

Pyroxidone deficiency (vitamin B6)

Pyroxidone is necessary for the conversion of tryptophan into serotonin which is a neurotransmitter which, when deficient, can cause depression.

Oestrogens can cause depression due to their impact on serotonin metabolism. Therefore, it is quite likely that those women using hormonal contraception are at an increased risk of suffering from depression. Any disturbance of tryptophan metabolism may result in anxiety, depression and a lower sex drive. An impairment of glucose tolerance may also occur.

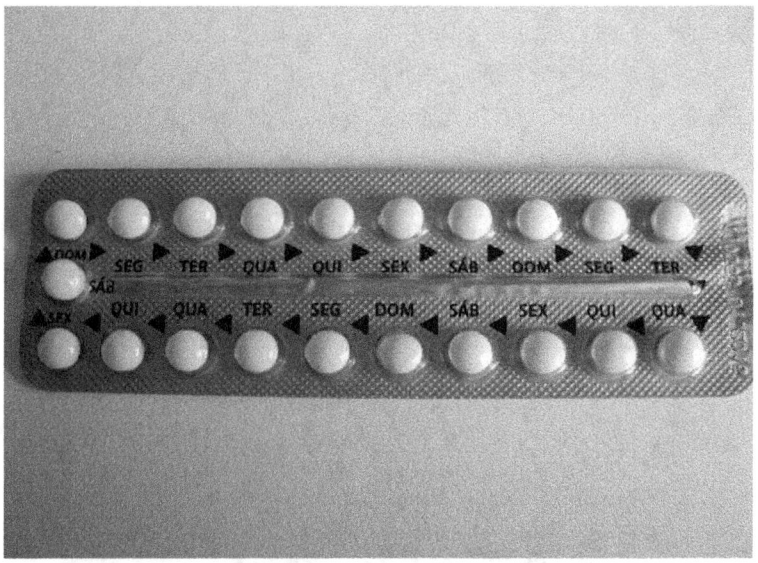

Contraceptive pills can interfere with pyroxidone and cause depression.

The normal intake of pyroxidone should be 100-500mg daily but when 40mg of Pyroxidone was given therapeutically then there was mood improvement as it was able to restore biochemical values.

Indication of pyroxidone deficiency may be considered if the patient also has a chronic reddish scaling inflammation of the skin. It is often found in cases of psoriasis, rosacea and acne.

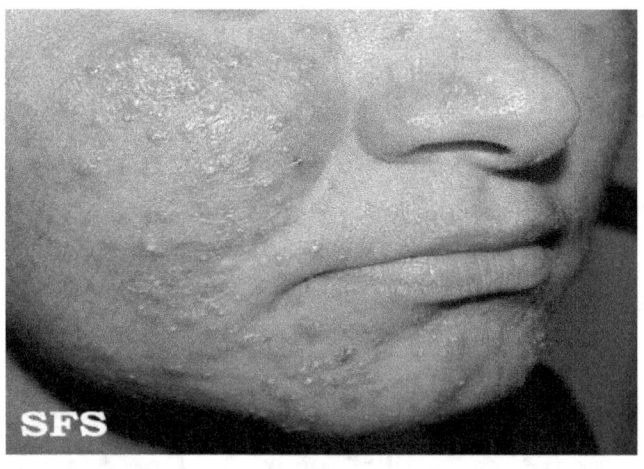

A typical skin condition that may be found with a pyroxidone deficiency in adult

Good food sources of pyroxidone are:

Beef liver, tuna, salmon, fortified cereals, chickpeas, poultry, bananas, cantaloupe melon, dark green leafy vegetables and oranges.

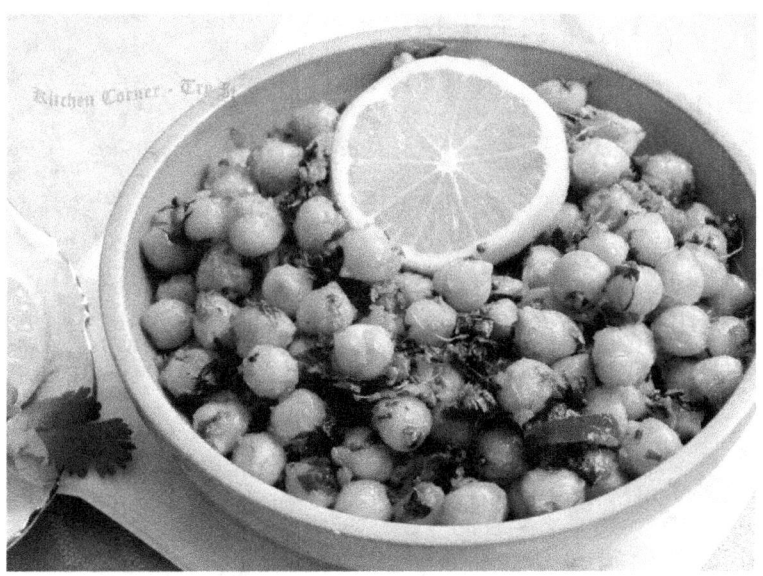

Chickpeas have useful amounts of pyroxidone in them.

Apart from hormonal contraceptive devices, depression due to pyroxidone deficiency can be induced by drugs and premenstrual tension. If drug induced, it requires at least 25mg of B6 daily to treat this condition. Premenstrual tension may need 50mg to 100mg from day 10 of the menstrual cycle.

Further indications that you may have a deficiency of pyroxidone are: anaemia, kidney stones and atherosclerosis.

Conditions such as asthma, urticaria, convulsions and mental retardation all require higher than recommended daily intakes.

Pyroxidone has therapeutic use in morning sickness, travel sickness, bronchial asthma and skin allergies. Any of these and the above mentioned conditions should alert you to the fact that a pyroxidone deficiency may be present.

In addition, further deficiency symptoms include splitting of lips, inflamed tongue, migraine, irritability, breast discomfort, swollen abdomen puffy fingers and ankles.

The B complex are all water soluble and many are degraded easily by light, heat and cooking. When food is cooked in water or steamed, the B vitamins will leach into the water and generally be thrown away. You cannot always depend that the amount found in food will be the amount available at the end of food processing or be wholly bioavailable to the body. The B vitamins are vulnerable in many respects but their impact on mood disorders can be life changing.

Given that B supplementation is generally low cost and the results life changing, it makes sense to try this highly efficient but long forgotten treatment.

Such is the nature of affective disorders that many people do not believe that relief can be obtained for condition. It may take general encouragement from others to aid motivation to at least begin to try some of the remedies in the book. Some may respond to this and others won't. I think it is always helpful at the very least to have available foods to hand which contain many of these life changing nutrients. The beneficial change that you are wanting to see may take a little longer than the more concentrated nutrients found in supplements but it is a step forward in the right direction.

Vanadium toxicity

Vanadium is and essential trace element for chickens and rats! There is some discussion that it is also essential for humans. When a deficiency occurs in rats it can cause an upset in iron metabolism as well as inhibit growth in cartilage, teeth and bones. In addition, it can increase cholesterol levels and blood fat levels.

Vanadium in the form of vandate ions inhibits the sodium pump found in cells. These ions appear to mimic the effects of insulin insomuch that it can reduce blood sugar to hypoglycaemic levels.

Vanadium is able to cross the blood brain barrier and is therefore effective at reducing any desire for food. However, vanadium must be taken in very small amounts as it will damage kidneys.

Excessive vanadium, on the other hand, leads to a type of manic depressive psychosis. Vitamin C is able to remove excessive vanadium.

Most of the dietary vanadium is not absorbed although between 100mcg to 300mcg is probably ingested daily in a normal diet. Only a little is retained in the liver or bones.

Sources of vanadium are:

Food	Mcg/100g	food	Mcg/100g
parsley	2950	gelatin	250
lobster	1610	Fish bones	240
radishes	790	strawberry	70
dill	460	Calf liver	11-51
lettuce	280	cucumber	38

Vanadium has been found to inhibit sodium, potassium and ATPase activity which has been found to be reduced in depressive illness.

An experimental study[14] found that vanadium toxicity is associated with depression and sadness.

The B vitamin, biotin. (coenzyme R/vitamin H of which the natural form is D-biotin).

Although biotin is often associated with hair strength, a deficiency has been found to cause depression which is very similar to the symptoms found in a vitamin B1 deficiency.

A case report[15] found that a patient on total parenteral nutrition developed, depression, nausea and vomiting, paraesthesia, lethargy, headaches and insomnia.

---

[14] Witskowska, D, Brzeninski, J. Alteration of brain, noradrenaline, dopamine, and 5-hydroxy-tryptamine levels during vanadium poisoning. Pol. J. Pharacol. Pharm. 31:293-8, 1979
[15] Levenson, J L., J Parenteral &Enteral Nutrition, 7 (2): 181-3

After supplementation of 300mcg of biotin daily symptoms improved and the patient returned to his normal state.

In an experimental study[16], four normal subjects received a diet which was deficient in biotin only.

10 weeks later they suffered from fatigue, depression, anorexia, nausea, myalgia and sleepy. In addition, they had anaemia, paraesthesia, dry skin and hypercholesterolemia.

One of the best sources of biotin are found in:

Dried brewer's yeast

Wholegrains/wheat bran/wheat germ

Corn

Fish

Meat

Rice

---

[16] Sydenstricker VP et al, Observations on the 'egg white' injury in man. JAMA 118;1199-1200, 1940

Pigs liver and kidney

Yeast extract

Biotin deficiency does tend to be rare but there is a protein in raw egg white called avid in (an antimicrobial protein) which if raw egg white consumption occurs on a regular basis will cause a deficiency of biotin as it binds tightly to biotin so that digestion is inhibited.

Deficiency symptoms include: persistent diarrhoea, depression, nausea, smooth pale tongue, hair loss and loss of reflexes as well as the symptoms mentioned previously.

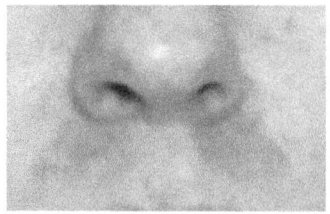

Periorificial dermatitis seen in those with a biotin deficiency

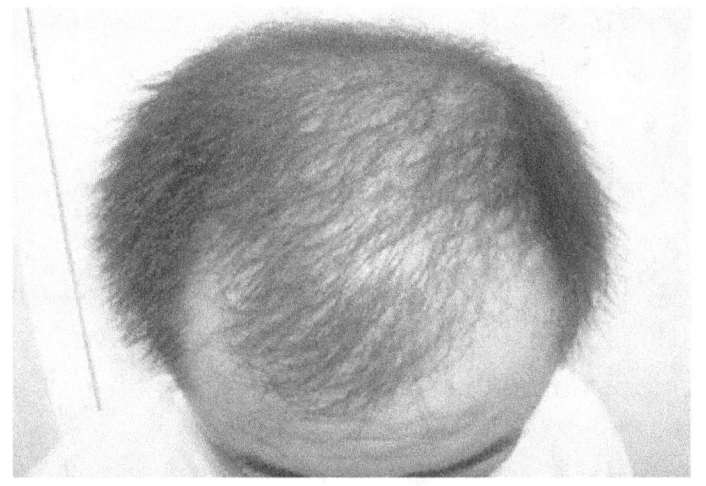

Biotin deficiency and hair loss

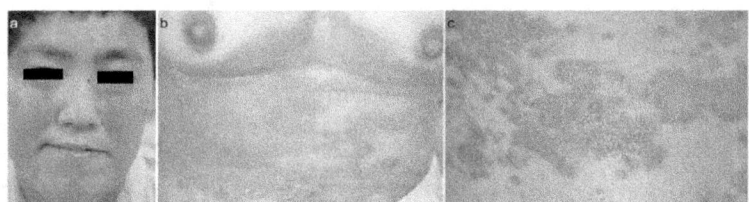

Signs of biotin deficiency

Iron deficiency

Iron exists as ferric iron or ferrous iron. It is an essential trace mineral which is found in the adult body at approximately 3.5-4.5g.

Most of the iron is found as haemoglobin which is the red oxygen carrying part. The rest is stored in the liver, spleen, bone marrow and muscles. In the muscles it is known as myoglobin and this stores some oxygen in the fibres.

The ferric form of iron is known to destroy vitamin E so if supplementing, the form of iron used in the supplements needs to be investigated.

Haem iron is found in meat and does not need vitamin C for its absorption. Non-haem iron which is found in plants does require vitamin C for its absorption.

Depression is part of the syndrome and is commonly found in women of menstruating age. Iron must be in the ferrous form to be absorbed.

Chronic deficiency is associated with depression and is generally the last sign to be corrected, once haemoglobin levels have been restored to correct levels.

In children, iron deficiency can also impair growth.

Low plasma levels of iron can also cause generalised itching which is also referred to as pruritus. This tends to occur more in the elderly than those younger but that does not mean it occurs only in the elderly.

Pallor in those with iron deficient anaemia is immediately noticeable. They look as though all the blood has been drained out of them. They are tired, lack stamina, breathless, have headaches, insomnia, palpitations. If you pull down the lower lid of their eye gently, the normally thin bright red blood vessels are pale, almost pink, suggesting a diagnosis of iron deficiency.

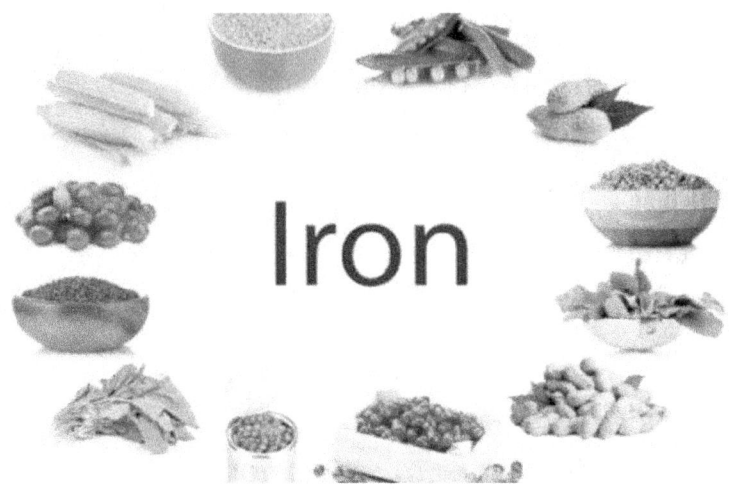

Vegetarian sources of iron.

The best sources of iron are the haem – meat sources – which are superior in that they do not need additional vitamin C for it to be absorbed.

Iron is known to dysregulate the bowel and pregnant females, who are generally given iron supplementation, will complain of the constipating effects of iron tablets.

Further, some bacteria will use iron which helps their replication so if an individual has an infection it is not always in their best interests to continue taking the iron tablets until as such time as the infection has gone.

The best sources of haem iron are cooked liver, kidney, sardines, corned beef.

As non-haem-containing plants come with their own vitamin C built in, it is tempting to think that iron absorption will not be a problem. However, vitamin C is easily destroyed by heat and light so there may not be much left once a meal has been prepared to enable the absorption of iron.

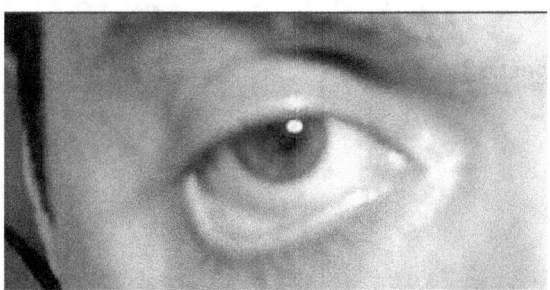

Note how pale the inner lower eye is due to iron deficiency anaemia.

We have now come to the end of the book but I wish to say this. Any book will only be able to cover a small amount of the infinite range of things that can impact on mood. Sometimes, we can pinpoint a problem fairly easily by the signs and symptoms associated with a particular deficiency or toxicity but it is not all plain sailing.

In this respect eating a varied diet in the company of those who matter to you will do much to alleviate the feelings of anxiety and depression that affect much of society now.

Thank you for purchasing this book. Every time a book is purchased, a donation is made to one of the charities I am currently supporting. Details of this can be found on my author's website.

Other Health Related Books by the Author include

- **The Reluctant Bowel**
- **A Weighty Issue**
- **Sleep, Perchance to Dream**
- **The Journey: EDS and chronic pain**
- **The MND diet: using nutrition to slow down the progress of neurodegeneration**
- **A Necessary Sorrow**
- **Treat infection Naturally**
- **Successful Aging**
- **Taking another Road: Pain: its causes and what can be done about it**
- **Osteoarthritis and Pain**

- **A Treatment Strategy for Migraine**
- **The Metabolic Syndrome Diet**
- **The Anti Virus Diet – only available through an independent stockist through Amazon UK only**
- **The Lipoedema Diet**
- **The Lymphoedema Diet**
- **Parkinson's Disease: dietary changes that work**

And many more

These can be found here on the author's page

https://www.amazon.co.uk/-/e/B07BPQZ5CD
and on Amazon worldwide

You may also be interested in the semi-autobiographical trilogy of the authors life found in these three books

- The Prejudged
- Where the Blackbird Never Sings
- A Summer's Symphony

And the author's children's books
- Fanny and Victorian Jack
- Fanny and the Gamekeeper's Cottage